Is ECT Right for You?

A "Friend to Yourself" Resource

By Sana Johnson-Quijada, M.D.

© Copyright 2014 Sana Quijada

All rights reserved. No part of this book may be reproduced or transmitted in any form or by any means, electronic or mechanical, including photocopying, recording or by any information storage and retrieval system, without written permission from the author, except for the inclusion of brief quotations in a review.

ISBN-13: 978-1499135701

ISBN-10: 149913570X

For more information about this book, visit http://friendtoyourself.com

Names, situations, and stories herein are the product of the author's imagination. Any resemblance to actual persons, living or deceased, is wholly coincidental.

For my brother, Vance Johnson, M.D.

Contents

1	At the End of Ourselves	1
2	The Value of Me	5
3	The Courage to Try	11
4	What is ECT?	19
5	Age and Reputation of Treatment	25
6	Who Should Consider ECT?	31
7	Staying Power and Maintenance	41
8	Conclusion	47
	Letter	49
	About the Author	51
	Disclaimer	53

Chapter 1

At the End of Ourselves, At the End of the Rainbow

Briggs was crying again. His wife, who came with him to our first appointment, looked like a peeled fruit sitting beside him. I could see she was undefended, giving her last layer of herself without knowing what would be left.

Briggs was the one with a case of serious depression, but his wife seemed worse off – heartbreaking. I suspected both of them, in their own ways, would not last long.

It is not unusual in a specialty psychiatric clinic like mine to work with people like Briggs. They have been around to all of the other treatment shops, and finally, in Jane Eyre style, they appear at my door "in the company of death."

They have been through therapies, practitioners, and churches, but disease can resist treatment, and they have not responded adequately. They have not healed. Everywhere they walk, it is as if Hades were visiting. It feels like hope-blossoms wilt as they pass by, and those of us who share their space feel like the ground is going to open up and suck us under. It is not uncommon in specialty care to be told, "I have no strength to go further." Like Jane, they plead, "I must die if…"

(By the way, Charlotte Bronte is the bomb.)

As the person on the other side of this exchange, I have a rainbow of "specialty" options available to offer. Yet some people, like Briggs, have not found relief, no matter how hard they try.

The human body and mind are not entirely predictable. Not every patient responds to the same kinds of treatments. Not every person follows a traditional path. Briggs and his wife were doing everything they could, but relief eluded them.

But there was one thing that they had not yet tried, and that one thing would end up making all the difference.

If you are here, reading this book, it may be because you are in a similar situation. You may think you

Is ECT Right for You?

are out of options. You may feel as if no one can help you.

There might still be a treatment for you.

Or perhaps it is not you walking through the shadows. Perhaps, like Briggs' wife, you came to this booklet because someone you love is suffering. You are desperate for answers, feeling helpless to change an illness that has taken over your own life, as well as the life of one you love.

You are not out of options. The journey is not over. You can still elevate the quality of your brain health. By reading this book, by seeking another opinion, by scheduling a meeting with a new specialty provider in your area, you continue to show levels of self care and bravery that must be applauded. By knowing there is a problem and being open to explore specialty care options, you are claiming your own need.

I am honored to share your company. You are a person of courage. Keep on!

Questions:

1. What brought you to this book? What are you searching for?

2. What treatment options have you tried so far, and what were the results?

3. Is there any treatment you think is too extreme to consider for brain health?

Please tell your story.

Self-Care Tip: Claim the need to find your specialty care.

Chapter 2

The Value of Me

The room is dark; the shades have been drawn for hours. Sandra stays trapped in her blankets. Around her, she knows there are gathering piles of laundry and stale air. Pictures have fallen over in their frames. Sandra hears her daughter pleading, "Mommy, please get up now. Let's get up, Mommy. I want you to get up."

Sandra's body feels like a bag of concrete, and she tries to explain to her seven-year-old, "I'm just so tired, honey. You go play."

Days, and then months, go by like this. Sometimes Sandra is up and functioning, but just barely. Her thoughts are not clear. It is hard to find words, let alone anything around the house.

"Who is this person?" Sandra thinks about herself. She wonders if her husband will leave her. Sex dwindles. They do not talk, and she is pretty sure she has not had a real orgasm in a year. She cannot believe he even likes her when she dislikes herself so much.

Sandra is not treating anyone very well because she has lost the sense of her own value.

It may not seem like a very posh thing for her to celebrate, to speak of, or to put at the front of the line, especially in this condition, but Sandra is worth it.

We are all worth it. You are worth it.

You are valuable.

Other things in your life—your status, your emotions, your perceptions—may change, but this will not. You are valuable. Spending time with you, even if only in your thoughts, is an immense privilege. That is true for anyone, including yourself.

You? Privileged to spend time with yourself? Yes.

Have you ever lost control of yourself? Have you felt the heat of anger hit your face as your thoughts fly into a rage and words rush out as if exploding dynamite? Bewildering, isn't it?

You know, then, what it is like to lose yourself.

Have you forgotten where your car keys are, but you don't care because you're still in bed and have no motivation to move? Your fingers, which once tapped socially across your keyboard, are idle now. Your calendar holds no interest. You hide, ashamed, because you just do not want to explain yourself to others. "It takes too much energy," you think.

You, too, know what it is to lose yourself.

It doesn't have to be this way. Being with you is a privilege, even if you don't know it any more. Reconnecting with your individual "Me" is a critical part of your health.

All those feelings and reactions you despise can actually be reminders that you are precious and of immense value. You are the reason people crossed the prairies, fought against the sun, and hunted for food to survive. You are the reason Noah's Ark survived for forty days and forty nights. You are the reason precious metals are considered lovely. And it is because of you that you want to be your friend. You are valuable.

But Sandra is having trouble accepting this. She's missing more and more work, and she's worried she will be replaced. "Who are these people?" she wonders about her focused, ambitious colleagues, the people she used to enjoy, joke with, and compete with.

Finally, Sandra realizes that everything worth living for is only insecurely hers. She is about to lose it all—her home, marriage, employment, possibly parenting rights. Her kids, her husband, her job—if she loses them, she thinks she will die. She needs to get better. She wants to get better. All the way better, back to herself: funny and sexy and showered. That would be nice.

Sandra takes what, for her, feels like a desperate action. She goes to see a psychiatrist. She tries to understand the treatment options described to her: medication, psychotherapy, and stimulation therapies.

In considering her choices, Sandra's doctor helps her think about how long it takes to respond to treatment; a patient's chance of responding to treatment fully, not at all, or only partially; and possible side effects. In Sandra's case, the situation is already dire. She needs something that works, and that works quickly. At the same time, she is suspicious of side effects. She does not want to gain weight or trade one set of medical problems for another. (We call these iatrogenic, when a medical treatment causes another disease.)

Considering this, Sandra decides that her best option is electroconvulsive therapy (ECT). Knowing that ECT can be up to 90% effective in reducing the severity of symptoms,[1] she starts her index treatment even before she starts having hope.

Sandra takes the one action she is able to toward her value.

---

[1] Bailine, S.H., Berstein, H.J., Biggs, M., Fink, M., Husain, M.M., Kellner, C., Knapp, R., Malur, C., McClintock, S., Mueller, M., O'Connor, K., Petrides, G., Rasmussen, K., Rummans T.A., Sampson, S., Smith, G. & Yim, E. (2000). Continuation electroconvulsive therapy vs pharmacotherapy for relapse prevention in major depression: a multisite study from core. *Archives of General Psychiatry*, 63(12), 1337-1344.

Sandra is not the only patient to reach for ECT when they come to the end of themselves.

In the previous chapter, we talked about Briggs and his wife. They didn't like the condition they were in, but because they valued themselves, they sought my help. While I was taking their histories, I asked for Briggs' medication history: medication names, when he took them, why he took them, for how long, why he stopped, and what they did for him. The list he gave me was long and comprehensive. Briggs had been at this for a long time.

I started thinking about numbers and percentages. I felt the foreboding.

Now, I am not a number person. (In the Jungian Typology, I'm a "big fat F" for feeler.) But even I could see that Briggs had been through a lot of trials and had tested almost everything out there. Nothing had helped.

Briggs was risky. He could die.

In Chapter One, I asked, "Is there any treatment you think is too extreme to consider for brain health?" I didn't ask Briggs directly, but that day I wondered about his answer. Briggs was courageous to fight the cruel sun the way he was. He was, in my eyes, why freedom and fresh flowers and hope remain. He was valuable.

"Briggs, what do you want to do now?"

He was valuable, and the next steps were his to make.

You are valuable, too. Like Sandra and like Briggs, you are the only person who can choose your self care. Your Me—your identity, soul, and self—is valuable, and being with you is a privilege.

Like Sandra and Briggs, your choices start with recognizing the value of Me and being willing to do what you need to do.

Questions:

1. If you are lost, what are you willing to do to be with yourself again?
2. How has recognizing your self-value increased your freedom to choose?
3. How has recognizing your self-value helped you decide what to do when you were or are ill?

Please tell your story.

Self-Care Tip: Remember, you are of value.

Chapter 3

The Courage to Try

As a psychiatrist, I have an arsenal of treatment options available to help the people who come to see me. One of the most controversial, and yet one that I am most passionate about, is the one that Sandra chose: electroconvulsive therapy.

ECT is not the right option for everyone, of course.

For one thing, it comes with quite the stigma.

You may have a clear picture in your imagination of ECT, built up from what the media has depicted. You may see a gurney with crisp white sheets and smell bleach. You may feel the long, quiet, foreboding ride toward the swinging operating room door, see the suspicious sideways glances of other patients and staff, and see the flickering of the fluorescent light in the hall. Does it make you want to turn and run? Take a peek at the patients around you. Are they like you? Do they seem better? Will this work?

Many of us remember Jack Nicholson's dramatic performance in *One Flew Over the Cuckoo's Nest*. It was graphic, painful, and memorable. But it was also a movie. ECT has changed and improved in the decades since then, when, admittedly, ECT was not much more than sticking your finger in a socket and getting voltage in a continuous sine wave for therapy.

ECT had a controversial beginning, and then lived in the shadows for decades. What stories emerged were scary. (Just search YouTube for "ECT stories" or "electroconvulsive therapy" to see what I mean.)

The truth is not nearly as dramatic. ECT is generally harmless. Modern treatment rooms are filled with staff members who love their jobs, because there is immense gratification that comes from assisting with healing. Patients fight for themselves each morning they set out for ECT, and they do it because it works.

Many people see ECT as a last resort, an extreme option for dire treatment failures, because those are the only stories we hear. There aren't widely trumpeted statistics about how many people choose ECT, or how it helps them in comparison to or in combination with other treatment options. We do not talk about how ECT is a top-ranked treatment option for brain illness. (Many people use the term "mental illness" versus "brain illness," as they find it easier to accept that "my psyche is sick" rather than "my brain is sick." I use brain illness in this, just by personal choice, but you can use either interchangeably.)

The truth is that there are many people receiving ECT every day, but so little has been heard.

Come out, come out wherever you are.

Have you tried ECT? Has your loved one? The stigma perhaps made you hide your own experience, and I can understand why. ECT patients often report feeling judged by others, even more so than patients who are treated with medication or talk therapy. Although the only way to overcome stigma is through education and empathy, no one wants to challenge it alone.

And so ECT stays in the shadows.

I was driving the other day when a seriously cool veteran went cruising by on his Harley, about fifty American flags affixed in mysterious ways to his bike and person. I cannot figure how he held it all together, but those flags were not going anywhere he was not.

I had forgotten it was Veterans Day, even though my kids were all off from school and properly running amok. This man, in his leather skins and industrial number of stars and stripes, reminded me why. As we approached each other from opposite sides of the street, I saw him nod to another biker passing by. It was enough to say, "Hello. You are not alone. I am not alone. We connect by this brotherhood."

I watched him in my rearview mirror, and as soon as I got home I dialed my dad. "Happy Veterans Day," I told the man who had served in two wars in the Air Force. And I remembered: my patients who have served, my family who marched in the Bataan Death March, my own freedom. And I remembered that I am not alone.

We are not alone.

Sometimes we don't wear our history as confidently as that cool vet. How messy that would be, right? Or not. Imagine a world where people used their hard-earned losses as a tool to empathize with themselves and others. Where we could receive nods, not judgments, and accept the applause of empathy, as it may be. Transparency turns the tables on trouble.

But we do not use our losses or gains so well. This is why I think so few of us speak up about what electroconvulsive therapy has done. There's no one celebrating the hard-earned gains of these patients. There's no one using their stories to build a community of positive good will. The pharmaceutical companies and the media makes sure we hear about the miracles of medication therapies from first-person reports (heck, even second, third, or tenth-person journal studies). But who is responsible for sharing the miracles of ECT?

Today, an ECT seizure lasts only around thirty seconds. There are no broken bones. No tongues bitten through. There are no chickens sacrificed on anyone's chest. One of my patients, initially nervous, laughed when she realized that she would be anesthetized for an upcoming colonoscopy for much longer than she would be in an ECT treatment.

That's something that's rarely mentioned in ECT's reputation.

When I meet with patients to discuss their treatment options, I tell them about the physician who had undergone thirty-six ECT treatments (three index courses) himself, as a patient, and whose morbid melancholia resolved to the point where he could return to practicing medicine in full capacity. It's an encouragement for the patients, but I wonder: Why would the physician tell people about his history? What kind of recognition do you think he got when he returned to medicine? Were patients willing to go to him for medical care? What about the gamers, computer programmers, parents, husbands, young adults, the nurses or anyone from the functioning, productive public who had the courage to fight for themselves by choosing ECT?

There are plenty of questions. My patients often have concerns. You have concerns. There are reasons for concern.

Is it shameful being connected to that history?

You know what to do with shame.

There are few medical specialties that gather as many opinions as psychiatry. And there are even fewer medical treatments within psychiatry that draw so many frothing opinions as ECT. No wonder patients are quiet. No wonder we are concerned. What a target we would make if we spoke out.

So although we veterans of ECT perhaps have not spoken up, although we may not tear up at ceremonies for what our courageous self care has done for our country, or received thanks for how we fit in, although we may not hang flags or tattoo it into our skin, the ECT community is full of courageous, important heroes. Maybe we are not as cool in leather, but like that veteran, we are where we are because of those who have come before us. We have suffered and died and lived, and we are connected. We have community and we are not alone.

You are not alone. If you are in treatment, or have been in treatment, or are considering ECT, I encourage you to speak out and tell what you know. There are many of us who would benefit from your education and empathy.

Write down questions you have. Share them with someone: your online support group, your physician, your significant other, someone. Go to http://friendtoyourself.com/ and use the Contact button to share with me. I would love to hear your story.

Is ECT Right for You?

Questions:

1. If you were to tell others more about your medical treatment choices, how do you think they would respond? How would your honesty change the stigma around mental health treatment?
2. How do you celebrate what others think is shameful but you know is not?
3. What have you found about yourself when you confront someone else's negative opinion?
4. What has understanding your place as part of a community done for your ability to celebrate?

Please tell your story.

Self-Care Tip: Don't let stigma be a barrier in your willingness to receive treatment and to connect with others. Instead, celebrate your courage for seeking a better Me.

Chapter 4

What is ECT?

We have talked about reputation, stigma, age, and courage. But you may still be wondering about the basic information: what is ECT? How does it work?

Electroconvulsive therapy is a refined brain stimulation medical treatment that works by changing how different parts of the brain communicate with each other. Using electrical currents applied directly to the brain, ECT "turns down" those areas that have overactive connection and ups those areas that are too quiet.

These effects are similar to how medications work for brain illness, but since ECT is not chemically ingested, it often works without the same side effects.

For a long time, we knew that ECT worked, but did not have studies demonstrating how. As technology has caught up to the treatment, we now see electricity stimulate to elicit a seizure that, in turn, activates neurons throughout the brain and changes chemicals associated with brain health, including serotonin, norepinephrine, GABA and glutamate. These actions result in a decrease in the symptoms of mental illness.[1]

ECT starts with what we call the index treatment — around four weeks of ECT dosed generally three times a week, for a total of nine to twelve treatments. It can be administered in either inpatient or outpatient settings.

Outpatients visit a surgery center, similar to where medical patients go for a colonoscopy. Once they are checked in, a nurse helps the patient settle onto a gurney. Patients don't have to change their clothes. An intravenous needle administers fluids: first for hydration, and later, anesthesia once the procedure has started. Patients do not experience physical pain associated with the treatment, nor do they remember it.

After a patient is asleep, the psychiatrist uses a machine to deliver an electrical current, which causes a controlled seizure. The seizure lasts, in most situations, less than a minute. Usually in contemporary treatment, ECT is "unilateral;" that is, stimulus is administered only on one side of the brain

---

[1] Ballenger J.C., Burt T., George M.S., Goldman J., Husain M.M., Lisanby S., Marangell L.B., Nahas Z., Rush A.H. & Sackeim H.A.. Vagus nerve stimulation: a new tool for brain research and therapy. *Biological Psychiatry*. 2000 Feb 15;47(4):287-295.

Is ECT Right for You?

and in brief stimulating pulses, which decreases reported memory and cognitive-related side effects that plagued early treatments. (We will look more at possible side effects later in the book.)

Before beginning an index treatment, patients who are eligible for ECT must consider the costs, both to themselves and their caregivers. A patient will need transportation to the surgery center several times a week during the index trial, and they may not function at their optimal levels during those index weeks.

But every treatment has some kind of cost. Stopping medications is the top reason that patients relapse in brain illness. Medications must be remembered, often several times a day, and refilled regularly. Patients frequently self-sabotage their medication compliance with their shame, which they must confront every day when they are prescribed to take pills.

The true measure of success for ECT is in the numbers: 78% of ECT patients report a higher quality of life at six month follow-up.[2]

To understand quality of life, I want to introduce you to Marcos. He had always been a small man, and now his lines were wizened, his moguled nose sloped over a deep philtrum, and his ears flew like flags on the sides of his head. Looking at Marcos

---

[2]Baker, T. (2013, April 15). ECT can restore quality of life for some severely depressed patients. *GRU News*. Retrieved from http://news.gru.edu/archives/8402

was a study of human terrain. For someone who was so active and visible when seen by others, it was an apparent contrast to understand how disconnected he remained emotionally. Brain illness had harmed Marcos. It was as if he had been scooped out in places.

Marcos and I worked together for ten years in psychotropic and psychotherapeutic remedies, with only partial treatment responses that curved up on currents of hope toward an imagined healthy baseline. His improvements never reached a point where he would call himself "well," and too soon they drifted down despite our cumulative efforts.

Marcos was losing hope about the time I traveled to Duke University for an updated training on electroconvulsive therapy (ECT). I had just opened up a new outpatient ECT surgery treatment center—the first in our area—and I was encouraged by the possibilities.

When Marcos and I discussed ECT as a new option for him, he wanted it without contest. I still remember the way he leaned back in his chair that day in my office, almost animated for a change. His scrubber eyebrows were like punctuation marks around his eyes. "Yes. I want it."

Now, three years after he started ECT, Marcos' wife tells me he is better than he was on their wedding day. He is more connected with her, and their sex life is having a run. He is more connected with their kids, and everyone feels like he has become a giver. The kids' grades are even getting better. They both think he is closer to that baseline for brain health he never thought he was going to get. By taking care of himself—by taking time, courage, emotional energy, and even a ride to and from ECT—Marcos has discovered a new quality of life.

Quality of life is a term many people use to quantify general well-being, including concepts such as freedom, human rights, and happiness. A person's "quality of life" is a state of mind, not a state of health, which is uniquely perceived by that person. They are the things that describe what we think when we ask, "What makes life worth living?"

Marcos could not read before ECT; his concentration was too poor. Now he is reading everything he can get his hands on, from personal biographies to scientific articles. He has become an advocate for his treatment choices. With improved focus and attention, he perceives his memory is better. He believes he is interesting because he is interested in himself. He is more aware of how others see him and smiles back when he catches the looks he gets just by wearing that face.

ECT is not a cure, but it is a treatment option toward brain healing, better quality of life, and improved interpersonal connections.

Questions:

1. Did anything about the fundamentals of ECT surprise you?

2. How does ECT compare with your current treatment?

3. What are the costs of you current treatment (in time, resources, side effects, etc.)?

4. How would you describe your current quality of life?

Please tell your story.

Self-Care Tip: Consider your treatment(s) as a way to improve your health and improve your quality of life journey.

Chapter 5

Age and Reputation of Treatment

The older I get, the more reputation I accumulate. I am an old rug.

Have you ever seen a child – their smooth, unblemished skin like marshmallows; their eyes, cupcakes (my children's are chocolate); the way they look at the world open-mouthed, swallowing flies; the way the world looks at them? Both sides hungry.

We say, "They have it all," especially in contrast to us "old property." The truth is, they seem to have it all because they haven't been around for very long. They do not have a bunch of mistakes accumulated, crafted, and woven into their lives.

However, even the most innocent children only have a limited supply of beginnings. Even though each of us has the freedom to start over at any point in our lives, once we have been around, starting over doesn't mean going back to the beginning. These "first times" that the children are experiencing now will change their constitution, and eventually they, too, will be weighted with experience.

Experience is not a bad thing, though. There is nothing like working with a veteran staff member who knows how to do everything that my medical office needs. That person is different from somebody just out of high school—their experience gives them perspective and wisdom. And there is nothing like having a physician who has practiced for ten or twenty years, who has seen patients walk out angry, has seen patients die, has seen in person which treatments do what. And there is nothing like a pharmacist who has worked with a medication long enough to know the inside of it; that there are benefits and side effects, and when you cannot unravel those from treatment, you try to see it together. The office staff person, the physician, and the fresh child have experience, and those experiences are often reflected in their reputations.

Those who have been around longer take up more ink.

A treatment can be like that, too. The longer it's been around, the more experience it collects, and the more reputation it has.

It is like being at a party and seeing somebody familiar. You recognize her as the first to come and

Is ECT Right for You?

the last to leave at every party you've been to before. You've seen her hurt people and been hurt, and you recognize the swarm of gossips surrounding her. Even if you've never met her personally, when you see that person, you think, "Here comes trouble!" or "Yes! The party girl is here." Whatever it is, you've got to acknowledge that she brings something to the gathering. She's lasted a long time, and there is a reason she keeps getting invited back.

Treatments are much the same way. A treatment that has been around for a long time, even when it has gotten a bunch of heat during its lifetime, has remained in circulation for reasons worth knowing. It's not a fad or gimmick. If it did not offer lasting and unique benefits, if its benefits were not considered greater than the risks and potential negative outcomes, if people's lives were not improved more than they were damaged – that treatment, like so many others, would have extinguished on its own much earlier in history.

ECT has been around for eighty years.

That is a big deal.

Every couple weeks, it seems, physicians and office medical staff thrill at a new medication sample. Salespeople deliver shiny, colorful boxes, well marketed with TV commercials and approved by the FDA, with the hope that we will be inclined to add it to our prescription roster. And it works. Physicians are happy to pull out their medicine cabinet drawers and present patients with the latest treatment, and with it new hope.

But what do we really know about a new medication?

A medication patent may last up to twenty years, with exclusivity for only eight years. Most medication trials in the United States study medications on hundreds or thousands of people over several years, but only for about 8-12 weeks on any one patient. The decision to launch a medication is based on the results of complicated mathematical statistical analysis. Once it is on the market, researchers continue to collect data, which is made transparent to the community.

What will we discover about Medication X over time? Maybe nothing dangerous or intolerable. How about eighty years? Medication X might remain in a safe category. Or maybe not.

During pharmaceutical trials for psychotropics, meaning medications related to brain health, the outcomes and treatment responses are often compared to patient reaction to ECT, which is the "gold standard" and baseline to help us understand our expectations. It has the longest, most consistent reputation in modern medicine.

The program for releasing medication is not a bad system, and I am grateful to be a part of the community of physicians who studies and prescribes medications from this pool of treatment options. Still, it is worth noting that despite the huge number of persons who received Medication X, none of them individually received the study drug for very long.

That's not much time to build a reputation.

Eighty years has its own kind of luminescence.

You with reputations, who are older than this and still around, tell us your story.

Questions:

1. How does the age of a treatment (or program or activity) affect the way you see it?
2. What do you think when you look at a treatment that your doctor offered you? Does reputation matter? Do you consider how long it's been available?
3. Research the history of any medication or treatment you are currently taking. Has it been offered long enough to get a reputation?

Please tell your story.

Self-Care Tip: When considering treatments, consider their age as you consider their reputation.

Chapter 6

Who Should Consider ECT?

Electroconvulsive therapy is not for everyone, of course. But it is an important option for patients who are looking for a treatment to quickly, safely, and effectively treat brain illness.

ECT is useful for multiple brain illnesses, most commonly mood spectrum illnesses such as depression and mania, and mood-associated problems such as psychosis, suicidality, and in some anxiety conditions.[1] These illnesses destroy our lives in many creative and tragic ways.

ECT starts working in one to two weeks, versus medication therapies that can take six to eight weeks.

---

[1]Tharyan, P., & Adams, C. (2005). Electroconvulsive therapy for schizophrenia. *The Cochrane Database of Systematic Reviews*, doi: CD000076

The speed of efficacy with ECT can be life-saving for a person who is deeply struggling. "Timing is everything," they say.

Quickly addressing brain health also brings long-term benefits:

- Patients experience less dementia, or cognitive decline, than individuals with untreated brain illness. Depression, for example, is associated with an increased risk of subsequent dementia when untreated.[2]

- Patients experience fewer impacts of other brain illnesses, which can emerge when one brain illness is not fully treated. A person experiencing a current illness is more susceptible to other problems, and more likely to let them go untreated. And ECT (as with medication therapy) done earlier in an illness episode has a more robust response; relapses are less severe, and a patient does not "drop" as rapidly when treatment is obtained quickly for a current illness episode.

- The faster that a treatment works, the sooner patients can start rebuilding their lives. Quick treatment can improve quality of life, halt the damage to interpersonal relationships, diminish financial challenges that are often secondary to disabling symptoms of brain illness,

---

[2]Jorm, A. (2000). Is depression a risk factor for dementia or cognitive decline? *Gerontology*, 46(4), 219-27. doi: 10.1159/000022163

minimize side effects, and minimize medications.

Of course, speed doesn't matter if a treatment does not work. When it comes to effectiveness, ECT works more often, more quickly, and more thoroughly than any other treatment option available to those who suffer many brain illnesses.

ECT is 20% more effective than medication at any point in a patient's treatment.[3] In other words, whether a patient is experiencing a first episode or fifth episode of brain illness, ECT is 20% more likely to get a positive treatment response than psychotropic medication. And treatment response is much more robust when ECT is combined with medication. Furthermore, patients suffer less illness relapse when ECT is continued in maintenance.

The primary reason for a patient's relapse in brain illness is medication noncompliance. A doctor prescribes a treatment, but then the patient fails to follow through. This is often related to the huge, pill-dotted elephants in the room: intolerable side effects and their cascade of related issues. Even dry mouth can lead to root canals. We risk osteoporosis from serotonin agents, or blurred vision, numbness, and tingling. Not to mention not achieving orgasm. And it's just hard to remember to take pills.

---

[3]Janicak, P., Davis, J., Gibbons, R., Ericksen, S., Chang, S., & Gallagher, P. (1985). Efficacy of ect: A meta-analysis. *American Journal of Psychiatry*, 142(3), 297-302.

Even the most diligent among us generally miss a dose or two.

ECT is easier to remember, and maintenance ECT is much less frequent than taking pills every day. Even when the ECT is combined with medication, if a patient misses a day or two of pills, the ECT is still likely to be consistent (offering prophylaxis against relapse), as it has the support of the community: the ECT staff and the transportation person to and from the surgery center.

In these regards, ECT has fewer barriers to treatment compliance that the majority of us suffer with medication therapies. That is a big deal.

But what about side effects? When I talk about ECT, curious patients often ask me about possible brain damage. ECT does not cause brain damage. It will not sizzle your brain, change your personality, or turn you into Frankenstein's relative.

And since ECT does not go through the body systems, it is not metabolized, and does not touch our organs. It does not affect metabolism, heart, weight, appetite, sex drive, sexual performance, cause dry mouth, vomiting, diarrhea, life-threatening rash, or any other common or bizarre side effects.

The side effects of ECT are best measured on an individual basis, as qualified by the person going through them. Important statistics and controlled studies show that the side-effects of ECT are generally headache and temporary memory loss.

During index treatment (the first three to four weeks), it is common to experience difficulty imprinting or recording new memories. This side effect usually disappears after about five weeks, and a patient's memory-making abilities return toward baseline. Eighty years of data do not demonstrate that there is other widespread memory loss, but there are individual reports of autobiographical amnesia, or memory loss.[4]

Public opinion of ECT, largely influenced by the media rather than data, has a very hard time believing that the memory loss is of new memories (or imprinting memories) during the course of the index trial – not memories before ECT, not memories after the index trial is done, not memories when maintenance ECT is going on.

After a seizure of any kind, whether artificially induced with an electrical stimulus or through pathology, the brain has a period of "quiescence." That is, it becomes quiet, and its natural activity rests and recovers. During this time, it makes sense that we will not imprint memories well. It's also typical for patients to feel sleepy, not remember events surrounding the seizure, and even possibly suffer disorientation.

The way I usually explain this to patients is that memory loss from ECT is related to mechanical issues. Think of a rain gauge. After it rains, we see

---

[4]Mudiwa, L. (2014, March 26). Media source of 'bad' portrayal of ECT. *Irish Medical Times*. Retrieved from http://www.imt.ie/news/2014/03/media-source-of-bad-portrayal-of-ect.html

on the gauge that it rained 2.3 inches last night. We uncork it at the bottom, and all the rain water flows out until the rain gauge is empty. We let the water out, and then recork it to measure the next rain.

To a brain cell, the electrical stimulus of ECT and subsequent seizure is like the process of uncorking the rain gauge. Everything that's there—in this case, the material inside the cell that we need to form memories—drains away. The brain then "recorks" after a stimulus, regardless of what causes it: pressure, magnetic, chemical, or in this case, electrical, and the cell starts to fill back up. When it's full, we can once again create new memories.

The stimulus and stimulus response do not damage the cell. They empty it, the way nature intended, and then it starts to refill. Until the cell has that inside content, it cannot lay down new memories. In psychiatry, we call this kind of reaction "mechanical."

The recorking process happens all the time in our brain after natural stimuli act upon a cell, be those natural stimuli pressure, magnetic, chemical, electrical, or other. ECT just intensifies the process. That's one of the reasons it's so effective: ECT is a medical therapy that uses the basic recovery methods of our natural physical design.

This explains why the memory loss is most often temporary rather than long-term. Cells replenish between treatments. The closer together the treatments are (and they are closest during indexing), the more the degree of memory loss. As the time between treatments increases, the recovery time also lessens, and so patients no longer notice memory loss. Their bodies are refilling their cells quickly after a stimulus, and they can once again imprint memories without difficulty. The rain gauge, we could say, has its cork in for longer periods of time.

Studies demonstrate, as does the collective opinion of anecdotal experience, that ECT memory loss is temporary.[5] Within a few weeks of the index treatment course ending, the memory returns to normal.[6]

Happily, most people say that within fifteen days of initiating ECT, their perceived memory is actually better than it was. This is likely because brain illness affects a person's perception of how they lack concentration and how they poorly remember things. The term to describe this kind of perceived memory loss is "pseudodementia." Some of my patients have complained during that time of memory so bad that they fear they are getting demented. In fact, they are depressed, not demented. Their memory is just fine, and when the brain illness brings healing, the symptoms of the brain illness (here, memory loss) improve.[7]

---

[5]Baghai, T., & Möller, H. (2008). Electroconvulsive therapy and its different indications. *Dialogues in Clinical Neuroscience*, 10(1), 105-17.

[6]Meeter, M., Murre, J., Janssen, S., Birkenhager, T., & van den Broek, W. (2011). Retrograde amnesia after electroconvulsive therapy: A temporary effect? *Journal of Affective Disorders*, 132(1-2), 216-22. doi: 10.1016/j.jad.2011.02.026. Epub 2011 Mar 29.

[7]Tsaltas E., Kalogerakou S., Papakosta V.M., Kontis D., Theochari E., Koutroumpi M., Anyfandi E., Michopoulos I., Poulopoulou C., Papadimitriou G., & Oulis P. (2011). Contrasting patterns of deficits in visuospatial memory and ex-

Headaches are the other common experience after the first couple of ECT treatments. After the first few treatments, personalized anesthesia medications are generally able to resolve these. (Not universally, of course, but generally.)

Once the transition from the index course to maintenance treatments evens out, memory loss and headaches are not common complaints from ECT patients, and other side effects are negligible.

But what about...

Pregnancy?

ECT is the gold standard when it comes to treating pregnant and peripartum women, because the treatment does not touch the organs, blood stream, or body systems that affect a fetus. In addition, it works, and it works quickly.[8]

There are no psychotropics that are considered "safe" for a fetus. Even serotonin agents that were once the go-to pills for OB-GYN physicians are now known to risk increasing bowel irritability, lung function problems, and heart disease.

Elderly patients?

ECT is the first line here, as well, for the same reasons – it is an effective treatment that does not

---

ecutive function in patients with major depression with and without ECT referral. *Psychological Medicine*, 41(5), 983-95. doi: 10.1017/S0033291710001443. Epub 2010 Aug 3.

[8] Miller, L. J. (1994). Use of electroconvulsive therapy during pregnancy. *Psychiatric Services*, 45(5),

Is ECT Right for You?

touch the body systems. As we age, medications metabolize differently, interact more, and can cause life threatening side effects. Even medications that a patient has taken safely for years can, one day out of the blue, cause dizziness and falls. It starts causing nausea. As if betrayed by an old friend, older patients' organs are sickened, and their health deteriorates via treatment efforts rather than improves.

Having a medical treatment that does not need to be metabolized avoids all of that.

None of this is to say that one person's choice of ECT treatment is superior to another person's choice toward a different treatment. Better or worse is an individual opinion, and each patient must do what's best for them, with informed consent. Rather, what I want to communicate is that ECT is under-utilized largely because of ignorance and stigma. Psychiatry is not an area of medicine with a huge array of treatment options. To obscure one of this caliber, with its life-saving, heroic, and life-changing import, is a huge loss. ECT is another paradigm of treatment. It is not an either/or, unless you want it to be.

Who are we to say who should risk experiencing the side effects of ECT rather than those of one medication or another? Only the patient can say how side effects compare against the benefits received from treatment.

Questions:

1. What side effects do you experience in your current treatment plan?
2. Are the side effects worth it to you for the benefits you're receiving?
3. Have your choices toward treatment ever changed based on dispelling your own stigma?
4. Has information and greater understanding of your treatment options ever specifically improved your self care?

Please share your story.

Self-Care Tip: Give deliberate consideration to both understanding and comparing the risks to your treatment and the benefits with other treatment options.

Chapter 7

Staying Power and Maintenance

From time to time, I hear complaints that someone's brain illness got better with ECT, but then came back when the ECT stopped. This almost always happens when a patient has not transitioned to maintenance ECT.

When my son was about one year old, he decided that if he turned his head away from you, it was as good as denying your existence. Turn. You're gone. Turn back. You reappear. Turn. Just like that, you have been eliminated. Every time he saw me it was as if I had appeared for the first time. Even now, remembering it delights me.

Not so cute, however, is disease relapse.

I call this the Tower of Babel Syndrome. At some point in life, we all make the mistake of trying to be like God. Or at least a lesser god. In this situation, after a patient has paid the price, after they have complied with the many hard tasks, after they have built themselves up into something glorious, they believe that they are cured from illness. They stop perceiving illness, and so they believe that being healthy, they are not in need of medical care. They are the gods of their own health, and don't need help. They fill their wings and off they go, living life free from disease-laden earth.

But this is a mistaken expression of freedom.

Sabrina came to our treatment center with her sadness, anxiety, and inattention in full swing. Six and a half months ago, Sabrina stopped ECT. She was going to see her primary treating psychiatrist, so she didn't bother to make appointments at the surgery center. The time slipped away. Now here she was.

She was able to say that she knew she could get better. However, her body and expressions all told me she was bewildered. She did not know that she could get better. She wondered who she really was and how this could be happening to her again. She was vulnerable.

The number one reason for relapse is treatment noncompliance, not necessarily life stressors. All those reasons for why we feel what we feel and do what we do, all those forces acting on us from

So how often, after the index treatment trial, after we feel healthy and behave well, is ECT necessary for maintenance? It depends.

After the index treatment is done, your doctor will taper the ECT doses down slowly, monitoring for symptoms of brain illness resurfacing. When you both decide that the symptoms are starting to come back, you'll stop the taper and continue ECT treatments at that frequency or a step before.

For example, if you recognized that your symptoms were resurfacing when you were getting one ECT treatment every three months, we would consider increasing ECT frequency to every two and a half months, and we would monitor to see that your brain illness remained fully treated. If you relapsed, we would increase the ECT dosing again until you responded fully, and then try to taper down again. These ECT adjustments can also be done parallel with efforts to taper medications as well.

Every patient is different in this area. Remember Marcos, from Chapter Four? After a year of treatment, Marcos had not been able to taper down ECT to less than one treatment every two weeks. We have tried many times, but every time we do his symptoms come back. He and his wife ask me separately and together, "Why? What's the point of decreasing treatments when they work so well and we're not having any problems from them?"

When we decide we want to go forward with treatment, we will be able to stay in treatment better the outside in, are not the reasons we relapse most often.

There is a super-bug growing amongst patients who engage in treatment on and off. I meet people who comply four or five months out of seven. They skip here and there, and they don't over-react when they miss an appointment or take a month off. "They don't control me, after all," is the attitude. Not being consistent with their medical treatment demonstrates their freedom.

Take treatment. Disease continues. Stop treatment. We are superior.

As noncompliance continues, and patients bounce back and forth, in and out of treatments, the super-bug starts to build, growing a super-resistance. The patient's number of falls into relapse accelerate, both in how long it takes to drop and how hard and far the fall is.

For most patients, walking away from treatment will not bring about freedom from disease.[1]

ECT, like other treatments for brain illness such as medications, is not a cure. Healing does happen, but the genetic predisposition of the illness is something that remains. Good to know, though, is that despite the time-line, maintenance ECT has a protective effect on the brain, reducing the chance of relapse when going through follow-up treatments.

---

[1] Fink, M., & Taylor, M. (2007). Electroconvulsive therapy: Evidence and challenges. *Journal of the American Medical Association*, 298(3), 330-332.

if we look inside and explore what we have in us that is pressing against the force to start or stay in treatment. Most of the time, the barriers to entry have to do with feelings of shame. Close to this are the difficulties that come from home culture, the opinions of those around us, and logistics.

Full Treatment Response:

ECT works alone, as does medication treatment and talk therapy. However, treatments work best when used together. We know that our goal is full treatment response—not to only improve the illness some, but to get full response to treatment and to allow for maximum brain health.

Leaving brain illness only partially responding to treatment equals leaving the disease to progress. The disease processes don't stop if left without full treatment response – they keep worsening brain health over time. When we fight for full treatment response, we are fighting to stop disease progression. We fight for our brain health at this point in time as well as fifteen years from now.

So whenever you are considering discontinuing or continuing treatment, make the decision as a team with whoever your team includes: your clinician, family members, friends, educational materials, and/or your higher power. Do not do it alone. Do it in consideration of what your treatment is bringing you now, and what it can bring, both good and bad.

Remember that emotions and behaviors come from the brain and are symptoms of brain health, not your stick shift or steering wheel. Remember you are human, made up of carbon matter. Be deliberate about your choices in treatment, not deceived into giving away your freedom to choose. These choices have life-long benefits.

Questions:

1. How does the perspective that emotions and behaviors come from the brain influence your commitment to your medical treatment?

2. Are you fully responding to your treatment?

3. If you could improve anything about your treatment response, what would it be? What is seducing you not to comply with your treatment? Do you feel like a victim to it?

Please tell your story.

Self-Care Tip: Push for full treatment response and figure out how to stick with it.

Chapter 8
Conclusion

Electroconvulsive therapy, as one of my colleagues says, may be the last miracle of medicine. It can be a first or fifth line of treatment and still be a potent tool in fighting many brain illnesses. It is quick, more often effective, and highly tolerated. Although it has been around since the 1930s, it has evolved to be a safe, modern procedure.

There is wonder in why we get ill and why we heal. Even with all the mystery, we are empowered by knowing our own value. We are not victims, even to our own biology, unless we choose to be. Our treatment toward brain health is one more way we can use our freedom to choose.

Choosing thus courageously in freedom, we find that we are able to have better quality of life, and more connection to self and others. As Marco experienced, so shall we also find that by taking, we become more of a giver; "taking time, courage, emotional energy, even a ride to and from ECT, Marcos took and then was able to give."

Should we all be so blessed.

Letter

Dear Reader, neighbor, fraternity guy, plumber, community physician, mother, Harvard graduate, retired investor, high school dropout, person,

Thank you so much for your work increasing community awareness of ECT and diminishing social stigma. Thank you for having a life-work, such as this, for obtaining a powerful voice that people want to listen to, and doing what you have done to get attention. Your influence, hard-earned, is collateral and that you spend it "here" is huge. I am so grateful.

It is difficult to work with community awareness and social stigma. We are not special in this difficult experience, of course, and know that the bummer feeling that "I am alone" in it is a distortion. We are special for more than our suffering and we are connected.

Thank you for your company and illuminating presence. Keep on.

Your own,

Dr. Q

About the Author

Dr. Sana Johnson-Quijada is a practicing board certified psychiatrist, a lover of books, a mom, a wife, and a huge fan of Starbucks (as well as local California coffee houses like Maui Wowi Paradise Coffee or Cafe Bravo.)

She is in private practice, specializing in outpatient clinics (in person or by tele-psychiatry, a developing area of remote psychiatry services using technology,) and ECT (electroconvulsive therapy). Dr. Q is also the medical director of the University and Magnolia Surgery Centers.

She never gets tired of talking about becoming a friend to yourself. To this end, she blogs at http://friendtoyourself.com, where she hears and shares the concerns and perspectives of self-accountable people in the trenches.

Disclaimer

Stories and details included here come from my imagination, and are not reflective of any patients. The characters are fictitious, not based on real people.

The information in this booklet is provided for general education. Nothing I write is meant to engage the reader in a doctor-patient relationship, nor should it be relied upon as a substitute for professional medical care. Consult your own physician for medical evaluation and treatment.

www.ingramcontent.com/pod-product-compliance
Lightning Source LLC
Chambersburg PA
CBHW032342200526
45163CB00018BA/2163